How to Survive Lung Cancer

A Practical 12-Step Plan

The guide I wish I'd had when I was learning

How to Survive Lung Cancer

A Practical 12-Step Plan

Michael Lloyd

Cover Art by George M. Bruestle

ISBN: 978-1-4357-0471-8

Published by Lulu.com

This book is dedicated to

Elizabeth

Acknowledgements

First of all, I would like to offer special thanks to my wonderful team of doctors, nurses and assistants at Dana Farber Cancer Institute and Brigham Womens Hospital, including my lead Oncologist, David Kwiatkowski, Radiologist Elizabeth Baldini, Nurse Oncologist Pam Calarese, Lisa Botelho, Mini, Natasha, Deborah, Marie, Michele, Douglas, Mary, Mittie, Ana, Lissette, as well as everyone else with whom I came in contact, either directly or indirectly, including Dr. Sternberg, Dr. Ahmed, Dr. Higgins and Dr. Kashpirovsky. I'd also like to thank all of my friends and family members with special mention to my sister Lynn and brother-in-law Nic who went above and beyond to make sure every detail was tended to. In addition, I'd like to thank Pamela A. Dutka for editing advice, my friend Nathan Shippee for our weekly healing sessions, my reflexologist Sue Selden, Danette and

Margaret who emphasized the importance of healing through forgiveness. Special thanks to Lexi, Lucy, Missy, Lee, and all my other friends and family members who gave me the space, support, love and understanding I needed to heal. I'd also like to thank anyone else I am momentarily forgetting to mention, and last but not least, I'd like to remember Eva, Rebecca and all others who have faced this illness courageously and are still with us in spirit.

Contents

Preface

In January of 2001, after almost a month of being sick with what I thought was the flu, I started to cough up blood. The diagnosis was an advanced case of small cell lung cancer, the fast moving kind with a large inoperable tumor in my lung that wrapped around my pulmonary artery and another tumor in my brain. I knew even before the doctors told me that my odds for survival were very slim. However, I also knew that I really wanted to live. I had no interest in hearing what most patients did. All I wanted to know was how the survivors had handled it. What did they do? What was their attitude like? What did they eat? What did the survivors have in common? To my surprise, the doctors I spoke to could not tell me. All they could do was quote grim statistics and recommend the conventional course of treatments.

The information in this guide is not meant to take the place of your doctor's advice. It is meant as a supplement to help clear up some of the confusion that you will encounter and provide you with powerful tools and direction to help you heal. There are additional references listed in the back including web sites that you can research on the Internet. However, the sheer volume of books and information available on cancer can be overwhelming and hard to digest especially when being faced with a diagnosis that is urgent and life threatening.

I've organized this book in 12 manageable steps. My goal is to help lung cancer patients benefit from my research into how other survivors beat the odds combined with my own personal journey developing the skills and knowledge I needed to overcome this illness. I explain in detail the specific techniques and exercises that I practiced on a daily basis to help me heal including ways to deal with issues such as fear and anxiety.

In retrospect, this is **the guide I wish I'd had when I was learning how to survive lung cancer.** I hope it inspires you to take a proactive approach in formulating your own magical combination to help you restore your mind, body and spirit to an optimum state of health.

– 1 –

Decide You Want To Live!

"Life is ten percent what happens to you and ninety percent how you respond to it."

Lou Holtz

The first and most important step to surviving lung cancer is to decide that you want to live! Everybody wants things but not everybody is willing to do what it takes. Just saying that you want to live is not enough. You must truly want to survive and be willing to do whatever it takes to overcome anything and everything that gets in the way. That's the attitude, first and foremost, that you need to succeed.

O⊸ The body reacts to our state of mind. Studies show that positive thoughts and emotions can produce positive chemical changes in the body. A fascinating example of this is known as the placebo effect, a phenomenon whereby giving sugar pills to patients who think they are receiving medicine can actually produce the same chemical changes in their body as those taking the genuine medicine. Just the fact that these patients believed they were receiving a medicinal cure triggered some sort of healing mechanism that effected the cure. Conversely, it has been shown that negative thoughts and emotions will produce negative effects on the body and can actually cause part of the immune system to shut down. Therefore, it is essential that you learn to maintain a positive attitude. It will physically help you to heal.

The mind/body connection is a very funny thing. You can cut yourself without realizing it and not feel any pain until you look at it. Then, all of a sudden it hurts because you believe it'll hurt and panic sets in. When it comes to cancer, try not to panic. It's important to recognize that every kind of cancer has a survival rate. There is not one form that is 100% fatal. So, even if the doctors say that the survival rate is only 2%, decide that you will be one of those two.

Refuse to accept any predictions regarding how long you have to live. They are only guesses based on statistics that do not apply to 100% of the cases. Again, keep in mind that every form of cancer has a survival rate. You must remain obstinate and decide to survive.

I once read a story about an elderly lady who was quite proper but when told by her doctor that she had a terminal case of cancer with only four to six months to live, looked squarely into the eyes of the doctor and said, *"Go f _ _ _ yourself!"* Asked when that was and she said over six years ago. She felt the doctor had a right to give her his diagnosis, but not to tell her how long she would live.[1]

Expect to Succeed

Numerous studies have been conducted with accomplished people from all walks of life, from successful business people to Olympic athletes, to people who overcome life-threatening illnesses. The most common characteristic found among them is their positive, winning attitude. Winners expect to succeed! This positive, winning attitude is more than just superficial backslapping. It comes from deep within. You have to truly

---

[1] Steven Locke, M.K., and Douglas Colligan, Foreword by Norman Cousins, *The Healer Within: The New Medicine of Mind and Body* (New York: Mentor, 1986) xviii.

believe you can do it and focus your mind like a laser on getting there. **O—** ***So, decide you want to live, expect to succeed and be willing to do whatever it takes.***

Staying positive in the face of adversity is not always easy and like most things in life, takes practice. To help, I recommend listening to motivational audio tapes on a daily basis. There are several tapes to choose from, dealing with a wide range of topics. Some tapes deal with attitude and others are specifically designed to help you relax and relieve stress. Others deal directly with healing. You may have to try a few different tapes before finding ones that you really like. It often comes down to personal preference and sometimes, it's just a matter of liking the sound of someone's voice.

Practice developing your breathing techniques with the following audio tape/CD, *Rejuvenate your Body/10 Minutes to Relaxation* series by Paul Overman, Ph.D. available through Barnes & Noble. In particular, listen to the track called *Body Scan* as often as possible to develop your skills. (More on breathing and visualization techniques later)

Louise L. Hay has made audio tapes that deal specifically with overcoming negative mental thought patterns that can be self-destructive. So when you are feeling somewhat defeated, listen to *You Can Heal Your Life - Audio Study Course*. She believes that deep hurt such as grief or resentment held over long periods of time can often lead to the onset of serious illnesses like cancer, causing the body to eat away at itself. She does a wonderful job of dealing with this by offering positive affirmations to help overcome these issues on her tapes and in her books. Louise also offers guided meditations in audio form that can be very helpful in learning how to relax.

Listen to *101 Power Thoughts* by Louise L. Hay in the morning. It will remind you of all the wonderful things to appreciate each and every day. Tapes like these can be listened to over and over again and will help program your mind to be more positive. I recommend reading any of Louise Hay's books as well, including her little blue book, *Heal your Body*.

Depak Chopra, on the other hand, combines an evolved spiritual approach with the metaphysical (beyond the physical) that is based in science. The stories he tells of patients he has worked with can be very inspirational. Read or Listen to *Quantum Healing: Exploring the Frontiers of Mind/Body Medicine.*

Visit www.hayhouse.com where there is an abundance of books and audio tapes/CDs by numerous authors that deal with mind/body approaches to healing. In addition, you can listen to a number of authors and speakers on www.hayhouseradio.com where they not only broadcast radio shows, but also archive old shows that you can listen to at no charge.

Even basic motivational tapes by people like Anthony Robbins can be beneficial and uplifting. Check with larger bookstores like Barnes and Noble or Borders where you will find a number of audio tapes and CDs available as well as a wide variety of books in their self-help sections. You can also check with your local library to see what they may have available in audio tapes/CDs and books.

I once worked in an office with a sign on the wall that read, *Attitude is Contagious. Is yours worth catching?* It was a nice little reminder that when you are in a good mood, people around you tend to be in a good mood. Happy people with a positive attitude lift the spirits of those around them. Unfortunately, the reverse is also true.

O━ *Be sure to surround yourself with positive people*. The last thing you need is to be around someone who is negative, always talking about doom and gloom. It will only bring you down which you simply can't afford, especially while in the early stages when you will need all of the positive energy that you can muster. If necessary, kindly have someone explain to them that you must put their relationship on hold while you heal.

We don't always have control over events that take place in our lives but we do have control over how we feel about them. There are people with very little in life who are happy and there are people who are healthy and wealthy but very unhappy. So it really depends more on attitude than circumstance. As my father once told me, *It's not how well you are ... it's how well you can live with the way that you are.*

From the moment I was diagnosed, I knew it was going to be a challenge and a grim one at that. Yet, at the same time, I felt it could also be viewed as a journey, an adventure that I was about to embark upon. Instead of hanging my head low and feeling sorry for myself, I decided to take as upbeat an approach as possible. Given a choice, I'd much rather be happy than sad, especially knowing that being happy and having a positive winning attitude would increase my odds for success and make my journey more enjoyable.

To add to my adventure, I bought a digital camera and photographed all of my doctors and nurses. I also took it with me on walks. When I told my sister about it, she asked if I had ever seen anyone else in the treatment center with a camera and I said no. I guess I was viewing it more as a holiday than a final destination. The following Christmas, I made copies and placed them in little plastic frames as gifts for all the wonderful people who had helped me, which made me feel good as well.

This book is filled with positive activities and various techniques that are designed to help you maintain a positive winning attitude. Take a proactive approach. Realize that you can greatly improve your odds for success through your attitude and actions. You don't have to take photos but you can find tapes that you like and allocate time to play them. You can't do everything at once, but you *can* do something at once.

– 2 –

Conventional & Non-conventional Medicine

"We only think when we are confronted with a problem."

John Dewey

The intent of this chapter is to discuss general treatment options, not to advise you on what to do. Ultimately, the decision is yours, and frankly, that is the way you should want it. After all, it's your life and you should want to play an active role in the decision making process.

Conventional medicine refers to what most doctors in America would recommend. Chances are, you will be sent to see a group of oncologists and their associates, doctors who specialize in treating cancer with traditional treatments of the day, such as chemotherapy, radiation, and in certain cases, surgery. Usually, this is where your journey will begin.

Non-conventional medicine includes everything from nutritional therapy to mind/body medicine, therapeutic touch, homeopathy, herbal and botanical, energy healing, spirituality, acupuncture, Qigong, etc. There are numerous articles and advertisements for these alternative approaches found in books and magazines at your local health food store and on the shelves of your local bookstore. There are also many web sites on the Internet with plenty of information and you can consult alternative practitioners such as naturopaths and homeopaths as well. In fact, there is such a large amount of information out there concerning various alternative approaches available that it can be overwhelming, and often, too much to sort out.

Multi-treatment centers are springing up that combine conventional with non-conventional treatments. More doctors are recognizing the effectiveness of complementing conventional medicine with additional care in areas such as nutrition, spiritual health and energy work offering, among other things acupuncture and Reiki. There is clearly a movement underway within conventional medical institutions as well that embraces these integrative treatments or what is also referred to as complementary alternative medicine (CAM).

Ultimately, I believe this is the wave of the future and hope we see more of this as time goes on.

Clinical trials are usually associated with conventional treatment/research centers that deal with up and coming treatments still in the testing phase. You can ask your doctors if they know of any you might qualify for that they would recommend. Be sure to ask about the advantages as well as disadvantages and look at how far along they are in the testing process, or what phase they are in. Just because a treatment is new does not necessarily mean that it is better. You may also find that different treatment centers are involved in different clinical trials, so it may be harder to obtain multiple and objective opinions. Nevertheless, they are worth asking about.

⊶ *When in doubt, do as the survivors do.*

According to Greg Anderson, leading researcher, author and founder of the Cancer Recovery Foundation, *most cancer survivors employed a combination of conventional and non-conventional treatments.* The vast majority of survivors integrated conventional treatments with a variety of complementary and alternative techniques.[2]

Since my case was so advanced, I decided to follow the advice, beginning with conventional treatments. However, before integrating non-traditional approaches, I consulted with my doctors to make sure what I did would not interfere with the conventional treatments I was undergoing. Researching and engaging in these complementary treatments gave me a sense of responsibility for my own health and well being. It also gave me a feeling of empowerment, being a part of the solution, not just part of the problem.

Every situation is different and what's right for one person may not be right for another. Therefore, all I can do is offer you ideas and suggestions to help you make the decision that is best for you.

There was a time when I thought I would never go through chemotherapy, but like many things in life, you really don't know what you would do until you are thrust into the situation. Just after being diagnosed, I read about a miracle

---

[2] Greg Anderson, *Cancer: 50 Essential Things to Do* (New York: Penguin Putnam Inc., 1999), 177.

cure that had occurred at an alternative treatment center in Chicago and I was able to get an appointment there for the following week. At the same time, I was trying to learn more about people who go to Mexico for non-conventional treatments, although the only person I knew who went did not survive.

If my case was not so urgent and advanced, I would have spent more time seeking additional alternatives, but I was being pressured by the first group of doctors I saw to start immediately with radiation to my brain. However, before doing so, I wanted to get a second opinion and since my diagnosis indicated small cell lung cancer (the fast moving kind) and it already appeared to have spread to my brain, there was no time to waste. I felt that I had to decide between going to Chicago where I could get more of a non-conventional opinion, which was more like a first look at an alternative approach or find the best traditional treatment center that I could find for a second conventional opinion.

Armed with the knowledge that most survivors pursued a combination of conventional and non-conventional treatments, and since it appeared that my life was in immediate danger, I decided to go the traditional route first, knowing I could follow with non-traditional alternatives. So, for a second opinion, I went to the best conventional treatment center in the region that I was able to get into, which was Dana Farber in Boston, about two hours away.

The doctors at Dana Farber, like my first group of doctors also stressed the urgency of my situation but they strongly recommended I start immediately with chemotherapy to my lung which was a distinct difference from what the first group of doctors wanted to do. Again, I would like to stress that every situation is different, but in my case, the first group of doctors I visited wanted to start right away with radiation to my brain and then combine it with chemotherapy, whereas the doctors at Dana Farber wanted to do the exact opposite by treating the lung first with chemotherapy and then, later on, treat the tumor in my brain with radiation.

When I told the second group of doctors what the first group recommended and asked *why* they wanted to do it in reverse, the main doctor (thoracic oncologist) looked me right in the eye and said, *because the tumor in your lung is much larger and will kill you well before the one in your brain, so we should concentrate our efforts on the lung first.*

He was blunt and to the point, but that is what I needed. There was no time to beat around the bush. Although it was pretty harsh to hear, I appreciated his direct approach. Plus, his logic made sense to me and I didn't have to be a brain surgeon to understand it!

I felt more comfortable with the doctors' approach at Dana Farber and they appeared to have more experience with my particular type of cancer. I followed their suggestion and within 48 hours began chemotherapy to my lung. It was an extremely difficult decision to make, but in retrospect, I truly believe if I went with the first group of doctors, I would not be here today.

– 3 –

Making Decisions

"It is not enough to do your best; you must know what to do, and THEN do your best."

W. Edwards Deming

From the moment of your diagnosis, you will be put on what I call the spinning wheel. Making a decision is not easy when the world as you know it seems to be spinning out of control. Here are a few tips that might help.

1 – Get a spiral bound notebook and use it to organize everything in one place. Keep a pen within the spiral binder so it will always be handy. I like the midsize notebooks (approximately 9.5" x 7") with section dividers that break it up. You can arrange the book any way you want, but basically, you will be writing down information to help you stay organized

and make better decisions. For easy access, use one of the section dividers or inside covers to write down any phone numbers that you need, like those of your doctors and nurses. You can also turn the book upside down and use the pages just before a section divider as a special place to write out your instructions for the pills you will be taking or to keep a list of your appointments. Use one of the sections as a daily journal and write down your observations, thoughts and feelings. Call it your wellness book and bring it with you to all of your doctor appointments.

2 – Enlist the help of a trusted friend or relative. If possible, have them come with you to your doctor appointments. However, make sure that you remain involved in the decision making process. That way you will be able to embrace your plan of action and increase your chances for success. Again, it is your life on the line so take an active role.

3 – Prepare a list of questions before meeting with doctors to get the most out of your visits. Ask about anything that you don't understand. Write the questions down in your wellness book and leave spaces for the answers. Do not allow yourself to become intimidated, even if you know nothing about

medicine. This is no time to worry about how ridiculous a question might sound. What would be ridiculous is if you were to allow these decisions to be made by someone else without understanding what you are doing and why. Remember, if you understand the decisions that are being made on your behalf, you can better support the plan of action which will increase your chances for success. Plus, no one knows your body as well as you do and what's right for you might not be right for someone else. So, if you feel that your doctor is not willing to explain everything to your satisfaction, you should seriously consider finding one who will.

If there is anything said that you do not fully understand, ask: *What does that mean? or... Why is that? or... Could you kindly explain that to me? or... Could you please repeat that? This is all very new to me, so could you please explain it in a way that I can understand?*

Each case is different and therefore, many of the questions you ask will be based on your specific case and on the course of treatments that your doctors recommend. However, here are some general questions that might help.

How certain are you of my diagnosis?

How many times have you seen a case like mine?

Does everybody treat it the same way?

What options do I have?

If you were me, what would you do? Why?

What other options do I have?

What else can you think of ?

Where would you go for a second opinion? Why?

What else should I know ?

I started bringing a voice recorder to appointments because I was not able to write down everything that was being said and my mind was spinning from the overall gravity of the situation. However, after a couple of visits, I found that preparing a relevant set of questions in my notebook and leaving a space to write the answers worked the best.

4 – Always, always get a second opinion. Get copies of scans and any lab work that was done and bring them with you. Doctors are used to it and insurance companies will pay for it.

Not only will you be able to double check your diagnosis and recommended treatments, but part of what you are looking for is the right team of doctors to work with. The better you feel about your team of doctors and your plan of action, the more you will embrace it and the better your chances will be to make it work.

Every case is different, but in my specific case, the lung surgeon I visited ruled out the possibility of surgery due to the fact that the tumor in my lung was wrapped around my pulmonary artery. Therefore, my main team of doctors that I had to evaluate consisted of the following:

1) Thoracic Oncologist (the head lung cancer doctor)

2) Radiation Oncologist (the doctor who specializes in radiation treatments)

3) Nurse Oncologist (the one who ended up being my closest contact overall, helping the other doctors and working with daily issues such as prescribing blocking drugs to help mitigate treatment side effects)

O→ You should try to get the best information you can from at least two different groups of doctors before making a decision and do not be afraid to ask questions to help decide who is best for you.

5 – Network… Contact anyone you can think of who could help you find the right team of doctors. Call any kind of doctor you know. Briefly explain your diagnosis and ask where he or she would go. Then ask them to call and make an appointment for you. This is no time to be shy. Doctors will often get an earlier appointment scheduled than if you call yourself, but don't be afraid to call different treatment centers on your own to see how they sound over the phone. Are they friendly, courteous and patient?

6 – Check out The American Board of Medical Specialties http://www.abms.org to make sure your physician is Board Certified. You can also call your State Public Health Department for additional information that may be helpful (see Additional References section at the end of this book).

7 – Try to be objective when weighing your options. Although it's not easy to make an unemotional decision when you are

emotionally upset, it might help you to write down the plusses and minuses on paper. Open your wellness book and draw a line down the center of a page. On the left side, write down all of the negatives. On the right side, write down all of the positives. After seeing it clearly written out in black and white, you may be able to look at it more objectively.

8 – Listen to your inner voice, your gut instinct. Let your conscious be your guide. We have infused knowledge that we can tap to help make a decision. You might try listening to the *Body Scan* CD (mentioned on page 4) and then, after being in a state of relaxation, think about your options. Quieting yourself in this way can help you to hear your inner voice. Some people say they know something in their heart, or feel it in their bones. Trust your instincts.

Emotions and Intellect

Even though I had intellectually made up my mind to begin chemotherapy within 48 hours of getting a second opinion, when it came right down to it, I was still unsure. I actually stopped and got out of the car as we were about to turn onto the highway heading toward the cancer center. I looked up to the sky and said, *what the hell am I doing?* Emotionally, I could not let go of the fact that I was going to subject my body to chemotherapy, something I had always been opposed to. Yet, if I let my emotions take over, I probably would have been paralyzed out of fear and not made any decision whatsoever.

Intellectually, I knew there was no time to waste. So, in order to keep moving forward, I continually reminded myself of how most survivors had employed a combination of conventional and non-conventional treatments and this was simply the conventional. Nonetheless, my emotions kept drifting to the thought of chemotherapy and how it would affect me, but when I put my emotions aside, I felt that given my specific set of circumstances, it was clearly the right thing to do.

My first day of chemotherapy started with hours of flushing my system with bags of liquids and pre-meds injected into my arm before they actually hooked up the chemo bag. As the time approached to start injecting the chemo, I knew I was about to poison my body. After all, the idea behind chemo is to kill the cancer cells, but I knew it would kill a lot of good cells too, something hard to be positive about. However, I also knew that in order to get the most out of the treatment, I had to somehow welcome this poison. As reported by the FDA, *"Expectation is a powerful thing... The more you believe you're going to benefit from a treatment, the more likely it is that you will experience a benefit."* [3] So I decided that if I was going to go through with this, I wanted to give it my best effort to make it work.

Fortunately, just as I was finishing up the liquids and pre-meds, and about to receive the chemo, a psychologist came by to ask how I was doing. As to be expected, I was scared. I told her my dilemma between my intellect and emotions. She asked me what each one said. Emotionally I was still afraid, but intellectually, I knew that I was in the best place for conventional treatments I could get into under the circumstances with a group of doctors whom I had the most confidence in. I also reminded myself that most cancer survivors employed a combination of conventional and non-conventional treatments. This simple exercise again helped me to reassure myself and added to my peace of mind.

---

[3] Robert DeLap, M.D., head of one of the Food and Drug Administration's Offices of Drug Evaluation.
http://www.fda.gov/fdac/features/2000/100_heal.html
FDA Consumer magazine / January-February 2000
"The Healing Power of Placebos"

So after deciding I was doing the right thing, in the right place, with the right people, I was able to welcome the poison just in time and breathe in a feeling of wellness as the chemo entered my bloodstream. I kept thinking of how this was going to help my body by giving it the boost needed to fight the cancer. At the same time, I would practice visualization techniques to protect my healthy cells and maximize the chemotherapy's effectiveness (more on this in Chapter 7).

– 4 –

Minimizing Stress

"Adopt the pace of nature, her secret is patience."

Ralph Waldo Emerson

Most doctors will agree that stress is the #1 underlying cause of illness. The APA reports that 75 to 90 percent of all physician office visits are stress-related and that stress is linked to the six leading causes of death.[4] Yet, conventional medicine tends to address the illness and ignore the underlying cause, leaving it to the patient to seek additional help to get at the source of the problem.

Stress can come in different forms. It can be caused by physical conditions such as inadequate sleep, poor eating

---

[4] *How Does Stress Affect Us?* American Psychological Association 2004
http://www.apahelpcenter.org/articles/article.php?id=11

habits, being out in the cold without proper dress, running up many flights of stairs, etc. Stress can also be of an emotional nature due to things like fear, making an uncomfortable decision, having a broken heart, feeling out of control, etc. Even good things can be stressful, such as getting ready to go on vacation or buying a new car.

The body can withstand an enormous amount of stress. The adrenal glands will produce adrenaline, providing bursts of energy that will allow the body to work even when it's sick and tired. However, if the stress is unrelenting and continues to build, the effects can be devastating. A very wise doctor once told me that deer can go through a difficult winter with very little food and many sleepless nights, as long as the spring comes.

It is unrealistic to think that we can eliminate all of the stress in our lives, but we can certainly minimize it. In fact, it's amazing just how much you *can* eliminate when your life is on the line. All of a sudden, things that seemed to be so important, no longer matter. Survival is everything, even when it comes to family and friends. If you do not survive, you won't be there to help them.

⚷ *One of the best decisions I made early on was to designate my sister to be my spokesperson.* I would tell her everything the doctors were telling me and *she* would tell the rest of my family and friends. She also did research on the Internet to see if what I was telling her made sense and we discussed any options I was facing. It took a tremendous load off of me. After all, how could I heal if I was going to spend a significant amount of time telling everyone how sick I was? It was just too stressful and all too real. I couldn't keep repeating what I was going through and still maintain a positive attitude.

As it turned out, not all of my family and friends were pleased with the concept of a spokesperson and I had to make a couple of exceptions but it was emotionally draining. I felt that every time I told the story to someone, it was just empowering the illness. This is not to say that I was in denial, but I just wanted to concentrate on my healing and visualize the positives, not continually relive the negatives. I was still alive and wanted to use all of my energy to figure out how to stay that way.

Receiving visitors was even more stressful. I could not help but want to look my best and would make the effort to do so, but it was exhausting. I had to learn how to limit the time and politely say that I really needed my rest before overdoing it. I even stopped reading my mail on a regular basis. The simple act of reading a get well card could make me want to cry. Old friends would recount meaningful moments in our past that were deeply touching, but emotionally exhausting and therefore very stressful. Although I greatly appreciated their thoughtful feelings and sentiments, I simply did not have the extra energy to deal with it at that time and I just wanted to stay in what I called: *My Wellness Zone*.

I was truly blessed with the woman I was with. Upon being diagnosed and having known each other for only four months, she dropped everything to take care of me around the clock. It was a huge sacrifice on her part. We created a wellness zone together and tried to make it fun as we embarked upon what I was determined to view as an adventure. She communicated often with my sister and also helped protect me from others by fielding any calls that were coming my way. *Above all, I cannot overemphasize the healing power of our love as she stuck with me through some of my darkest moments and I will forever be grateful.*

The next thing I did was to walk away from my business, a technology company I co-founded and was actively running. If someone had asked me if I could ever have done that two months before, I would have said absolutely not. No way! I was totally committed to the business and could not have imagined walking away. However, the work was very stressful and I knew *I'd have to do whatever it took* to minimize stress, including walking away with the possibility of losing everything I had been working on for years. I also eliminated all of my business e-mail so that I could devote my time to figuring out how to survive cancer with the same level of commitment I had devoted to my career. Fortunately, and because of my resolve, I was able to turn everything over to my partners with three phone calls, but again, that was because I decided that nothing mattered except staying alive. Period.

As for *physical* stresses on my body, I stopped smoking the day I saw the lung surgeon, and I dramatically changed my eating habits. I drank bottled water, stopped drinking coffee and did not consume any alcohol. I also stayed away from anything toxic that I could, including household cleaning products, gas stations, dry cleaning, second hand smoke, perfume and basically anything that smelled funny to me. I used Basis soap, which is very mild and washed my clothes with Dreft, a hypoallergenic laundry detergent made for babies.

Chemotherapy was enough of a physical stress on my body in and of itself. In my case, it was administered in three day courses with three weeks off between each course. It was a huge attack on my body that had a cumulative effect but the three weeks off helped me rebound.

I expected to experience a lot of nausea and vomiting during chemo but fortunately, advances in the field have made blocking drugs available that can eliminate most of the problem. I learned to work closely with my nurse oncologist who asked me many questions that helped her determine the right balance of drugs to mitigate side effects. I really only threw up once or twice that I can remember, but overall, the chemicals were really hard on my body. **⚷ *Make sure you drink an enormous amount of water as recommended, to wash the drugs out of your system.***

The biggest mistake I made was not taking it seriously when I first became constipated. With my body in a weakened state, becoming blocked felt like I was being poisoned. It led to a late night visit to the emergency room where fortunately, I was able to clear the problem with a Fleet enema. Needless to say, it was a memorable experience. After that, I paid attention to taking the right amount of laxative and stool softener on days leading up to and following the courses of chemo.

Here again, your wellness book will come in handy. Writing daily notes and observations on what drugs you take and when, as well as what side effects you are experiencing and how they appear to correspond with the drugs you are taking will help the doctors and nurses prescribe the right combination and dosages for you. There are a lot of things to coordinate and it's much easier and less stressful if you just keep a good set of notes as opposed to relying on your memory, especially while undergoing treatments.

The first week following a course of chemo was tiring, but by the second week I would feel better and began taking walks two or three times a day. The exercise helped to reduce my stress level and clear my mind enough to appreciate the life and fresh air around me. I didn't over do it, but I really looked forward to my walks. I would push myself little by little and extend the length each day. The moderate exercise seemed to get my blood flowing as well as my mind. It was during these walks that I began thinking about things I still wanted to do in life, all the things I had put on the back burner. It gave me more reasons to live and more resolve to fight the cancer.

You will have to decide for yourself what stresses in your life you can live without, or should I say live with by minimizing.

⚷ *Create a wellness zone and allocate your energy wisely.*

Remember, nothing matters if you don't survive, so give it your best shot and eliminate, or at least minimize every single physical and emotional stress possible.

– 5 –

Eating Well

"Let food be thy medicine, thy medicine shall be thy food"

Hippocrates

Eating well is one of the best ways to get healthy and stay that way. It is also a key factor in building up your immune system needed to fight the cancer. And it's not just *what* you eat but *how* you eat that can make a difference. Eating properly will help minimize the physical stress on your body, which, in turn, will help your body fight off illness.

To begin with, you should always consult your physician. They may have specific requirements and/or recommendations for your particular needs. However, many physicians often do not really know. For some reason, they don't view nutrition as something that is important enough to deal with. But more and more, doctors are becoming involved in nutrition or at least, will have a nutritionist on staff. If so, ask to speak with that person and see if they can put together a special program for you. Meanwhile, here are some general guidelines that I hope will be helpful.

One way to minimize physical stress on your body is to eat less but more often. Spread out the amount of food you eat throughout the day. This will help regulate your blood sugar level and won't be so hard on your digestive system. It is physically stressful to digest a large meal, especially when your body is in a weakened state. **⊶ *You are much better off eating six or seven snacks or small meals every two or three hours than to eat two or three large meals a day.***

Toxins

A great way to minimize the amount of toxins you ingest is to eat organic foods whenever possible. 'Organic' is the key word that you should look for. 'Natural' has no meaning. In order to become certified as Organic, the food has to meet certain requirements, for example, regarding the chemicals used in the soil.

Organic foods are not completely free of chemicals, but they are far less contaminated than their non-organic counterparts. Therefore, make sure to wash all of your fruits and vegetables, even if they are organic. Since many of the nutrients are found in the skin, get a little scrub brush to use with vegetables like carrots instead of peeling them.

Some people feel that organic foods are a waste of money. However, when your life is on the line, every little bit helps. Consider the fact that many of the chemicals used in commercial food production have been shown to *cause* cancer. It only makes sense that you would want to minimize your body's exposure to these chemicals, especially at this time. Fortunately, organic foods are becoming increasingly available in the major supermarkets and local farmers markets, and as a result, less expensive.

A healthy body can tolerate all kinds of toxic foods, full of preservatives and chemicals, but it taxes the immune system. Our bodies can even digest foods that we are allergic to.

However, it requires a lot more energy than necessary fighting these toxins and allergies at the expense of fighting off the cancer. So give your body a break. If you know of any food allergies that you have, try to stay away from them and feed your body the highest quality food possible. Again, the idea is to minimize physical stress whenever you can so that your immune system will have more energy to fight the illness.

Most nutritional diets and cancer diets in particular involve eating lots of raw fruits and vegetables. Over processed and over refined foods are of little nutritional value. Even cooking raw vegetables will destroy most of the vitamins and minerals essential to replenishing the body to its optimum state of health. Our bodies are living organisms and need live raw food to stay healthy. So, the question becomes, how can you maximize your intake of the essential nutrients found in raw fruits and vegetables?

☕ *Get a Juicer*

One of the best investments I made when fighting cancer was to buy a quality vegetable juicer. I bought the Champion brand, a heavy duty juicer built to last. More recently, I've used a Breville, which is a good brand as well. These machines are not to be confused with blenders or food processors. A quality vegetable juicer masticates raw vegetables, separating the juice of the vegetable from the fiber so that you can literally drink it, which is a far better way to obtain a vegetable's nutrients.

Juicing vegetables is almost like injecting live nutrients directly into the bloodstream. It gives you the maximum amount of nutrition with minimal stress on the body. When a vegetable juicer separates juice from the fiber, most of the nutrients stay in the juice, making it very powerful and much easier for your body to digest. Since virtually all food must become liquid before it can be assimilated, your body won't have to waste energy chewing and digesting to get at these nutrients.

Take for example, carrots, an anti-oxidant vegetable rich in beta carotene and known for its cancer fighting qualities. If you cook a carrot, you will lose most of its nutritional value. Even eating raw carrots, between the energy it takes to chew and the time it takes to go through the digestive system and into the bloodstream, you will have expended a substantial amount of its nutritional value. Whereas drinking fresh carrot juice will feed the maximum amount of live nutrients into the bloodstream within minutes and with the least amount of stress on your system.[5]

As for deciding on what vegetables to juice in addition to carrots, listen to your body. When I was going through chemotherapy, I would crave dark greens, like organic spinach, kale and parsley. I'd throw it all into the juicer along with a little apple or celery to sweeten it up. However, my daily favorite was a combination consisting mostly of carrots with spinach and parsley. If you are really in tune, your body will call for the things it wants and needs.

Fresh juice made from raw fruit or vegetables should not be confused with bottled juice that is bought in a store. They are not even in the same league. In almost all cases, bottled juice has been heated to increase shelf life, which destroys many of its vitamins and minerals. You would be better off just eating an orange or an apple than drinking store bought orange or apple juice.

In addition to their nutritional value, fresh fruit and vegetables

---

Dr. George H. Malkmus, *God's Way to Ultimate Health* (Tennessee: Hallelujah Acres Publishing, 1997) pp. 148-151.

are an essential source of fiber needed to cleanse the body. However, juice that is masticated in a juicer contains no fiber. Since fruit is easier to digest than vegetables, as a general rule:

⊶ *Juice your vegetables and eat your fruit.*

Juicing fruit is not bad for you. It's just that given a choice, eating raw fruit for your fiber causes less stress on your system. What I like to do is put whole fruit in a blender to make fresh fruit smoothies because a blender, unlike a juicer, retains the fiber. You do not throw the fiber away as you do with a juicer.

I made a lot of fruit smoothies with organic low fat yogurt and protein powder. My favorite, depending on what fresh fruit was available at the organic market, was made with a various mixture of bananas, fresh squeezed orange juice, a little apple juice, strawberries, blueberries, blackberries, red grapes, cantaloupe and any other organic fruit I could find. I would blend it in the morning and drink it throughout the day. Drinking too much fruit juice at once can cause a bit of a sugar rush and tax the body which will work against you, so drink it a little at a time without overdoing it.

You will also need a lot of protein as you head into chemotherapy and/or radiation treatments. I ate more eggs, meat and fish than normal, making a real effort to find the highest quality organics and antibiotic meat free of growth hormones as much as possible. I also ate a lot of organic legumes, nuts and whole grains. If you are worried about your figure, now is the time to let it go. Although I did not adhere to any specific diet, there are many special cancer diets and recipes available online and in bookstores. Health food stores often have books available and visit: www.amazon.com for the most complete collection of books on the subject. Just type the following words into the search box: *Cancer diet*.

In addition to eating high quality food, it is important to drink high quality water. My doctors recommended *at least* eight large glasses per day. If you do not trust your local water, drink bottled water. I chose to drink Poland Spring brand bottled water because I heard it's better than what some water companies offer. Drinking a large amount of water helps to cleanse your system, especially the kidneys, which really take a beating during chemotherapy, so drink as much as you can. Also, I like to drink my water at room temperature because it seems to be easier on my system and I did my best to exceed the recommended eight large glasses per day.

Before eating or drinking, take a few deep breaths. Quiet your body and think of the healthy nourishment that you are about to receive. Even when drinking water, try to visualize the cleansing effect that the water will have on your entire system.

A word on supplements

My doctors were adamantly opposed to my taking any supplements while going through chemotherapy and radiation treatments. They felt that some things could counteract with the treatments and therefore cancel out the effectiveness. The only things they approved of were taking a multi-vitamin once a day and drinking supplemental protein drinks to help maintain my weight. The rest of my vitamins should come from the food I ate. In spite of all the magical roots and cures I was reading about, I decided to stay on my current conventional course and learn how to get the most out of my diet. Again, I knew I could always follow with more exotic approaches or supplements later on if it appeared the conventional approach wasn't working.

Finally, you may decide to work with a professional nutritionist in order to create a custom diet that best suit your needs. If so, my favorite advice that I once heard someone say is: ***If you decide to see a nutritionist, find one who looks really healthy.*** ☺

– 6 –

Maintaining a Sense of Humor

"If you are going through hell, keep going"

- Sir Winston Churchill

I knew I was in trouble before I was diagnosed, from the moment I began to cough up blood. I also knew it was increasingly difficult for me to breathe. Then came the scared look in the face of the man who took my chest x-ray. If that wasn't enough, later that week as I was waiting to speak with the lung surgeon, his nurse said, *You mean they didn't tell you?* Her eyes were practically popping out of her head. Finally, the surgeon came in. A very somber man, dressed in a long overcoat, moving slowly but with precision. It was a very serious moment and I was there with a beautiful lady whom I had been dating for only four months.

The surgeon took my x-rays and carefully clipped them to his light box on the wall. He slowly pointed to a large tumor that was occluding my lung. He explained that it was wrapped around my pulmonary artery and said it was too advanced to operate on. *Great,* I thought. This was the first bit of good news I'd heard because I really did not want to get operated on. I didn't know how at the time, but I thought I'd just have to figure out another way to get rid of it. Then he said maybe they could shrink the tumor enough with chemotherapy to cut around my pulmonary artery and remove the whole lung, but even that seemed highly unlikely and it would greatly compromise my health. The best he could do was to prescribe a bottle of cough medicine for temporary relief and suggest I stop smoking.

Having just been confronted with the worst news of my life, I asked, *Can I still have sex?* He looked up and cracked a smile as he nodded. So I said, *Well then, I guess it could be worse.* I was pleased to get a smile out of him and even managed to get a little smile out of the lady I was with, albeit a painful one. I know it sounds crazy, but I was determined to look at the bright side and although I knew it wasn't going to be easy, I wanted to try and make it as fun as possible.

Humor can lighten up the most intense situation and I realized, at that very moment, how it would play a key role in the magical combination that I was developing to help me survive. I needed to be positive, and making a joke made me feel better, even if only for a moment. Plus, it helped diffuse the magnitude of the situation. It may seem a bit twisted, but it was actually easier than sadly facing the cold hard statistics.

I remembered reading a book many years before called *Anatomy of an Illness*, where the author, Norman Cousins was facing a life threatening diagnosis and basically laughed his way back to health. The doctors said his case was hopeless but he was determined to survive and decided to spend his time in the hospital watching Marx Brothers movies and old Candid Camera re-runs. His recovery was miraculous and it spawned a number of studies on the healing effects of laughter.

The American Cancer Society notes, *The value of humor has been confirmed to the point that many hospitals and ambulatory care centers now have incorporated special rooms where materials - and sometimes people - are there to help make people laugh.*[6]

---

[6] http://www.phoenix5.org/humor/HumorTherapyACS.html

As it turns out, laughing is one of the healthiest things you can do. It produces positive chemical changes in the body such as releasing endorphins that actually help boost the immune system. So look for something that will make you laugh. If you are going to watch TV, don't watch the news, find a comedy to watch. **⊙━ *Try to find something to laugh at, even if it's yourself.***

Another benefit to humor is that it can lift other people's spirits, which, in turn will lift yours. For example, advances in drugs make going through chemotherapy better than it used to be, but it's still not much fun. While being administered chemotherapy, patients are tethered to an IV pole, which is kind of like a coat rack on wheels. When you have to use the bathroom, which is quite often from all of the liquids, the pole has to come along. So you end up having all these people in the chemotherapy ward wheeling around their poles. I used to refer to mine as my dancing partner, like Fred Astaire dancing with his coat rack in the movies. The very thought of it made people smile, which, made me smile as well.

I actually felt sorry for my doctors because they had to deal with such morbid issues on a daily basis. How difficult it must be for them, knowing that the majority of their patients don't make it. However, I knew in order to survive, I could not buy into their worst case scenarios. I needed to be strong, but still wanted to keep it light. Sometimes, during an examination, I would lean forward, look intensely into their eyes and say, *I don't care what you find or where you find it, because I'm going to get rid of it... So there!* Then I'd lean back and smile.

Early on, I remember my doctor telling me that if I chose not to go through with the chemo, my neck would swell, my head would swell and then I'd die. I thought, hmmm… that sounds pleasant. Then, during my physical examination the nurse oncologist detected swelling in my neck which I could feel as well. It scared me but I knew I had to maintain a positive attitude so I tried to lighten up the situation with humor.

As I got up from the examination table, I reached out to touch the nurse's neck and said, *is your neck swollen?* Without thinking, she quickly grabbed her neck and said, *I sometimes worry about that.* Then she realized I was teasing and couldn't help but smile. At first, I'm sure the doctors thought my humor was strange, but as time passed and my health improved, we smiled and laughed together.

As I began each course of chemotherapy or radiation, I had to sign a form acknowledging the potential side effects of the treatments I was about to receive. These forms list all the terrible things that could happen. At first, the forms would really frighten me until I thought about the alternative, which was that I would die. So from then on, when I was presented with one of the forms, I would gasp and say how awful it was, pointing out the worst side effects and saying, *You mean this could happen?* Then I'd say, *but if I don't do it, I'll die, right?* Then I'd smile and say, *OK, I'll sign.* Here again, I found a way to turn a grim situation into one I could find amusing.

One of my favorites was another drudgery that I would turn into a game. It was when the time came for my periodic CT scans. There is no eating or drinking for 4 hours prior to the scan and when you get there, you are handed a putrid drink that makes you want to gag. For fun, I would thank the nurses very much for giving it to me and say, *You know I haven't had anything to eat or drink for hours, so I'm really going to enjoy this.* And the funny thing is, just saying that made it taste better. Then I'd make noises like *hmmm* and lick my lips while drinking it. Others in the waiting room would look at me and smile, knowing how awful it tastes. I'm sure some of them thought I was crazy but nevertheless, it brought a little cheer to not so cheery a situation.

I know not everyone is able to laugh about such serious matters and certainly, I wasn't always able to either. However, if you try to take a lighter look at these things you might find it reduces stress and makes it easier to deal with difficult issues. Plus, the added benefits of the chemicals that your body produces through laughter will help boost your immune system and physically help you to heal. So if you are going to go through it anyway, you might as well try to make it fun.

– 7 –

Breathing and Visualization Techniques

"Imagination is more important than knowledge"

Albert Einstein

While going through treatments, I used to playfully think, all I have to do is breathe and I won't die. It sounded easy enough. Although this was meant as a personal joke, it's a fact. All I had to do was keep breathing. Interestingly enough, the breathing exercises I practiced turned out to be one of my most enjoyable activities as well as one of the most important.

You can instantly calm yourself through breathing, you can monitor your state of health through breathing and you can heal yourself through breathing. **⊶ *When you combine breathing exercises with visualization techniques,*** *you will have access to an infinite source of healing energy that I found to be an extremely effective survival tool.*

If you have ever been involved in any type of yoga or meditation, you have already been exposed to breathing techniques. If not, just the fact that you are reading this means you are breathing, so it's just a matter of learning how to breathe for health.

Whether you are experienced or not, I recommend using relaxation tapes as suggested earlier. My personal favorite is called *Body Scan*, a track on the *Rejuvenate your Body/10 Minutes to Relaxation* series by Paul Overman, Ph.D. It starts out like most relaxation tapes, directing the listener to take slow, even breaths, at least 5 seconds or longer. While concentrating on your breath, the tape guides the listener through visuals of drawing your breath through different parts of your body, which can be used to relieve tension wherever it exists.

I prefer listening to this breathing tape on my back with my arms over my head which expands my chest cavity and lungs, allowing me to take deeper breaths. I actually got to the point where I could take in breaths as long and slow as 30 seconds, although I found 15 or 20 seconds to be just as effective. It takes a few minutes of listening to the track before I am able to take such deep slow breaths and it required practice but this is time well spent. In fact, of all the tapes or CDs I mention in this book, *Body Scan* is the one track I still listen to every day. I feel it helps me to overcome anything that ails me and it helps keep my mind, body and spirit in an optimum state of heath.

Very quickly you will realize that aside from feeling relaxed, you will begin to feel in control of your body and in turn, in control of your health. You will actually be able to direct your breathing to heal your body. The more you practice, the better you will get at it, and eventually, it will become a habit. Then, you will be able to do it anywhere and at anytime.

Monitor your breath throughout the day. If your breaths are short or if you are tense and you find yourself holding your breath, **⊶ *calm yourself instantly by taking deep breaths.*** Breathe slowly and evenly. Let go of the tension held in your face, jaw, neck and shoulders. You can close your eyes or just focus your thoughts inward. With each inhalation, silently say the words, *breathing is healing… breathing is healing…*

breathing is healing… You can also make long moans and groans as you exhale. These exercises feel good and can actually help you to relieve more tension.

Visualization

Visualization is a very powerful technique that is extremely effective when used in conjunction with breathing exercises, and the great thing is, you can do it anyway that you want. In other words, there is no right or wrong here, just whatever you can make work. I will tell you what seems to work for most people, and what works for me, but ultimately, the way to go is that which works best for you. So be creative.

A popular visualization technique used to break up tumors is to imagine the video game Pac-man as an agent to help you fight cancer. For those of you not familiar with this video game, it features an animated character that looks like a cracked eggshell moving through a maze, eating up whatever is in its path. What you do is visualize the Pac-man character eating up all of the unhealthy cancer cells in your body. Use your mind's eye to locate the tumor and picture Pac-man methodically seeking and destroying the cancer cells that are there. If you do not know where your tumors are located, ask your doctor to show you the scans so that you can better visualize where to concentrate your efforts.

Personally, I was never into video games but I watched cartoons as a child and preferred to practice this visualization technique using the character of Mighty Mouse, a Superman type figure with a cape. As I conducted my deep breathing exercises, I would imagine breathing in these healthy little Mighty Mouse characters that would fly into my lung and stamp out the cancer cells. I imagined them as my lifesavers. I could even hear the theme song in my head. It was the good guys against the bad guys. This type of thing may make you laugh, but do not underestimate its power. These visualization techniques will actually engage your body and mobilize your immune system to help with your fight against cancer.

At times, I would picture myself with boots on, stamping out all of the cancer cells, which I pictured as being weak and confused, versus my own strong and healthy cells. I would crush and grind the weak and confused cells with an image of my foot extinguishing them like cigarettes. Then I would kick them out of my body as I exhaled. Perhaps it had a double meaning, since I was trying to reverse the effects of my smoking. Again, use whatever image you like. There is no right or wrong here, just use whatever you can make work. Adapt these techniques and adopt them as your own.

⊶ *Practice these visualization exercises as many times a day as you can.* The more you do it, the better you will get at it and the more effective it will be. By continually practicing and developing your skills in this area you are taking control of your health and joining in the fight against cancer, not just relying on the treatments given to you by your doctors. The more adept you become, the more you will start to feel it working. Then, as you see positive results in your scans, become even more motivated to further increase your efforts.

In Chapter One, we talked about deciding to live, and the fact that everybody wants things but not everybody is willing to do what it takes. Here is a great example of where this applies. Some people will claim they don't have time to practice breathing exercises seven or eight times a day, yet, they will watch TV or talk on the phone for hours. It's a matter of priorities, and in my experience, you will have to make sacrifices if you want to give your body the best chance of surviving. Don't expect miracles to happen if you aren't willing to make any changes in your life.

Early on, I tried to be diligent and worked really hard on these techniques throughout the day and night. Then, when I was at the point where the doctors said that the tumor in my lung had diminished by 85 or 90%, I felt great about everything I was doing, but was afraid to lighten up because I really wanted to win this battle more than ever. So I decided to increase my efforts in everything I was doing.

O⊷ *Try ten times harder to get rid of the last ten percent.* As far as I was concerned, just having it on the run wasn't enough. I wanted to completely eradicate every last bit if it from my body so that it would go away and never come back. I increased the frequency of my efforts with passion and continued to work on creative visualization techniques in conjunction with breathing exercises, which, I still do in one way or another to this day.

As for the tumor in my brain, from the time it was diagnosed, I began using breathing and visualization techniques that I had learned many years before through biofeedback training. If you are new to all of this and are having difficulty relaxing through the CD's alone, you may want to give Biofeedback a try. It is non-invasive, fun to do and is proof positive that breathing and visualization techniques have a profound effect on relaxing your body.

Biofeedback teaches patients how to lower their stress levels through natural means, using their own capabilities. With the help of a trainer and equipment monitoring such things as muscle tension, pulse rate, skin temperature or brain waves, the patient learns techniques to quickly lower tension and control stress. The feedback equipment helps by allowing the patient to witness progress through the machine in real time, for example, lowering muscle tension as you are taking deeper breaths. Through practice, patients learn how to lower this tension without the feedback equipment and are able to incorporate these techniques into daily life.

In my case, I had learned how to use biofeedback to get rid of headaches by monitoring electrical activity in the muscles of my neck and shoulders. Through relaxed breathing and visualization exercises, I was able to lower the electrical activity in the specific neck muscles which relieved the tension that caused the headaches. Little did I know at the time how useful the skills I learned would become in lowering stress and muscle tension around the area where my tumor would be located. To learn more about Biofeedback, visit: http://www.holistic-online.com/Biofeedback.htm

I also used breathing and visualization techniques throughout my radiation treatments. As with my Mighty Mouse visualizations during chemo, I created various images to help increase the effectiveness of my radiation treatments and minimize any side effects.

Radiation treatments in my case, began with a day or two of setup work. This basically involved lying still while they designed custom blocks to focus the beam on my particular tumors and block the rays from hitting other organs unnecessarily. They even tattooed a few little dots around my chest area, used to line up the machine during treatments.

When the actual treatments started, they worked on my lung for a few weeks and then performed what is known as standard prophylactic radiation to my head. This is a common safety measure for most lung cancer patients to avoid the cancer from spreading to the brain. However, since mine already appeared to have spread, I agreed to have extra doses of radiation focused on the brain tumor itself.

The radiation machinery reminded me of a much larger version of an x-ray machine at the dentist office where everyone would leave the room before turning it on. Instead of a little click, each exposure lasted about 20 seconds and like an x-ray, you don't feel anything. The whole procedure only took about 20 minutes a day, five days a week, but in my case, went on for almost three months.

When I began each treatment, I'd try to relax with a few deep breaths and visualize breathing in pure healing energy to boost my strength. Then while the radiation gun was turned on, I would stay still and visualize the beam pinpointing any cancer cells that were left and disintegrating them with the laser type accuracy of a sharpshooter.

The cumulative effect of the treatments really tired me out, especially with the extra doses of radiation to my brain. To exercise my brain, I made use of the puzzles in the waiting room. After treatments, I'd sometimes sit and work on them for an hour or more. I found it to be a nice way to stimulate the part of my brain that deals with pictures and shapes more than words.

I believe that by persistently practicing breathing and visualization techniques, lowering muscle tension in my neck and exercising my brain with the puzzles, I helped my body achieve a successful outcome. In fact, I was initially told that brain tumors never completely disappear, they just become benign. However, I was pleasantly surprised a couple of years later, when my doctors said the tumor in my brain had completely disappeared. It was no longer visible and there was no evidence of disease! I joked and said I always knew there was nothing in my brain (meaning no intelligence) but what a miraculous outcome. Now, I can't prove it, but I really believe that the power of the breathing and visualization techniques that I employed helped to obliterate it.

– 8 –

Disposing of Fear

"The only thing we have to fear is fear itself"

Franklin D. Roosevelt

Fear is debilitating. In fact, it can paralyze you and totally derail your efforts to heal. We all experience it but when it comes to surviving lung cancer we need to learn how to deal with it. Even after successfully completing all of your treatments fear can continue to haunt you and undermine your efforts to stay healthy. Quite simply, you cannot afford to be slowed down by fear because you have too much work to do.

Having said that, I would like to say that fear is only natural, especially concerning cancer. Most people know someone who has died as a result of cancer and you may be experiencing a lingering fear of death. One of the greatest gifts I received from cancer that I cherish to this very day is that I am no longer afraid of death. Before cancer I was terrified of death. Now that I have faced it head on and learned how to deal with the *fear factor* I am no longer afraid, which is a huge load off of my mind.

In general, I think people are afraid of what they don't know. I found that some people are so afraid of cancer (the 'C' word) that they can't even talk about it. I was always afraid of a friend or loved one getting it but now that I've had it, the mystery is gone and I'm better able to deal with it. Plus, I really believe if your will doesn't break you can get rid of anything. Nevertheless, the fear factor was always lurking about.

The difficulty in dealing with fear is that it is intangible and very elusive. It is something that is hard to get your hands around. The best trick I learned that works really well was taught to me by an energy healer. We were discussing different visualization techniques that I had been experimenting with and she said if I relate better to visuals, put a face on my fear and then visualize disposing of it in a way that is harmless to others.

I immediately thought of a famous old painting called *The Scream*, depicting a horrifying face with a wide open mouth. I visualized plastering the face from the painting onto a Frisbee and throwing it away. As the Frisbee passes through my force field at the edge of my wellness zone, it gets shredded to avoid harming others. Now whenever I sense fear, I take a deep breath as I mentally plaster that face onto a Frisbee and throw it away while I exhale, letting go of any fear.

This may require a little practice, but don't worry, you will have plenty of opportunities. Fear has a funny way of creeping up again and again. However, this technique only takes about five seconds and you can do it over and over if you are being plagued. Simply plaster the face onto a Frisbee and throw it away. You will feel instant relief. If you are still worried, do it again. Take a deep breath and feel your shoulders drop as it flies away.

Another way to deal with fear is to do something constructive. This could be anything from going for a walk to eating healthy food. The idea is to make a positive move to distract your negative feelings. Play an audio tape, such as *101 Power Thoughts* by Louise L. Hay or read a book containing positive messages.

Do anything to change your thought pattern. There is a fun little book called *8,789 Words of Wisdom* by Barbara Ann Kipfer that I highly recommend. It is full of little sayings that will make you smile.

If it is fear of death that troubles you, it may be helpful to read about life after life. This won't work for everyone because not everyone believes in it but if you are open to the idea, psychic medium John Edward makes a compelling case in his book, *Crossing Over*, named after his television show. Another excellent writer in this field is world renowned psychic, Sylvia Browne. She has numerous books on the subject available through www.hayhouse.com. Again, this is not for everyone, but reading these books gave me comfort and helped me to overcome my own fear of death.

Here again, breathing exercises and visualization techniques can be helpful and quite calming. Think of a favorite memory or place you have visited such as your favorite beach or lake. As you breathe deeply, try to feel the gentle breeze in the air as you experience the sun shining down upon your skin, filling your heart with warmth. Remember what the fresh air tasted like and what the sand between your toes felt like. Can you remember what sounds were present? **O━** *Try to bring as many different senses to your visualization as you can while breathing deeply to make it feel as real as possible.*

Another technique you could try is sometimes referred to as grounding. This is where you stand on grass, with or without shoes, near a nice healthy tree. Breathe deeply and try to envision growing roots up through your feet, connecting you to the Earth. Continue taking slow deep breaths in through your nose and visualize pulling the air through your feet, right from the Earth. Ask Mother Earth to please bring up the white light as you breathe in the energy that heals us. Picture it weaving up through your body. Then, as you breathe out of your mouth, envision exhaling through your feet, emptying your fear and anxiety back into the center of the Earth. Ask the Earth to kindly take the fear from your body and dispose of it in a way that is not harmful to others. This technique is very effective and can produce instant results. It is a great way to boost your immune system and is something you can practice on a daily basis. I used to do it during my daily walks. It not only helps with fear, but also helps to balance your mind, body and spirit. When you are able to achieve this balance, you will feel at peace.

The same techniques that apply to alleviating fear can also help you deal with anxiety. However, if worse comes to worse and you cannot shake the feeling, it may be due to some of the drugs you are taking. I remember having problems with a certain steroid that I was given. Make notes in your wellness book including the time of day that the anxiety occurs and report it to your nurse oncologist. You may find that your anxiety corresponds with something you are taking. The nurse may also be able to provide you with other drugs to help overcome anxiety attacks. In addition, you can seek professional counseling if you or your doctor feels it would be beneficial.

Sometimes it's easier to talk about cancer with strangers than with a friend or family member. Support groups offer a great outlet for people who want to talk about what they are going through with others who are going through similar experiences. Although I loved sharing information and helping others when I went in for my treatments, it often saddened me and just added to my own fear and anxiety. So while I was still in the midst of it I felt a need to protect myself and preferred to stay in my own wellness zone.

If you are going to support groups make sure you are not getting sucked into what I call the doom and gloom of others. Mentally build a force field around your body to protect yourself from any negativity. Visualize your body inside of a bubble or pyramid, filled with healing light and energy. It's kind of like a portable wellness zone you can take with you. We actually exchange molecules with our environment so try to surround yourself with people who are upbeat and positive and try to stay away from those who tend to be sad or negative.

And last but not least, if you are really afraid, it should motivate you to do something about it like dedicating more time to breathing and visualization exercises. ⚿ *Turn your fear into determination and get busy!*

– 9 –

Energy Work and Integrative Therapies

"What is now proved was once imagin'd"

William Blake

Energy work and integrative therapies are continuing to gain acceptance throughout the modern western medical establishment, yet they are mostly based on ancient concepts. Often referred to as complementary alternative medicine (CAM), these treatments are much less invasive than conventional approaches to curing illnesses such as cancer. Although many in the medical community look at these therapies as a way to mitigate the side effects of conventional treatments, others consider these therapies to be legitimate alternative approaches to conventional medicine.

These complementary treatments and therapies include everything from Acupuncture, Acupressure, Reflexology, Biofeedback and Magnet therapy to Homeopathy, Energy work, Reiki, Qigong, Yoga, and work with Medical Intuitives, just to name a few. Wellness centers offering alternatives such as these are sprouting up across the country and even well established hospitals are bringing more of these therapies into the mainstream simply because there is increasing evidence that they work. You can find more information on these therapies in health magazines and on the Internet as well as through the additional references section at the end of this book.

With more and more integrative therapies becoming available, it can be increasingly difficult to know which one or ones to choose and why. How can you find the magical combination that will work for you? Is there a path that you should be following?

The answer in part depends on what ails you and where you are in the healing process. It might require trying a few different approaches or a few different practitioners of a particular therapy. For example, not all acupuncture practices are alike. You may even find that different treatments work on different ailments at different times. Like traditional medicine, it is not a perfect science.

Many of the concepts discussed in previous chapters, such as the power of positive thinking, visualization techniques, the mind/body connection, etc. come into play in various ways throughout most types of energy work and integrative therapies. They are organized differently but for the most part, are all based on the same underlying principles.

As I experimented with these progressive ways to help fight my cancer and its side effects, I realized that I had been preparing for this journey my whole life. I remembered as a student how I became fascinated with Eastern philosophies and psychology, not on the clinical side, but experimental psychology, and in particular, parapsychology, or beyond psychology. This included hypnosis, psychic phenomena and basically all of the unexplainable phenomena that did not simply fit into our current scientific world view. I experimented with meditation, studied Eastern religions, practiced yoga and read about psychic discoveries in the former Soviet Union. My goal was to find universal truths as yet undefined, by looking for common ground through cross cultural comparisons.

After graduating I continued my studies as a hobby. I read books on unconventional medicine that represented a broad overview of different practices from around the world. I traveled to churches where faith healings took place and visited mystery spots in Northern California where the earth appears to have gravitational warps. I was fascinated by electromagnetic energy and how it seems to intensify under pyramidal shapes. I even traveled to Egypt and climbed the Great Pyramid at Giza to feel the energy first hand, lying down in the sarcophagus early in the morning before other visitors arrived. I read old accounts of Atlantis, the Bermuda Triangle, and other odd occurrences. I trained in biofeedback and learned how to get rid of headaches, my own as well as others through the laying on of hands. I even learned how to dowse for water. What became clear through all of this was that the common thread connecting it all was an underlying universal force of energy that everything seemed to be utilizing, in one way or another.

I know there are a lot of skeptics when it comes to energy work and healers in general and I can understand why. With all of the fraudulent people in the field making all kinds of illegitimate claims, I'm skeptical too. In fact, I really have to experience something for myself before I believe it works and it has to make sense to me. I need to feel good about whomever I deal with or I won't even try it. However, when it comes to believing in the healing properties of this underlying universal force of energy, remember, just because we can't prove it as of yet, does not mean that it doesn't exist. In the early 1800's, before developing more powerful microscopes, we couldn't prove theories on the existence of germs or cells for that matter, which today are accepted in everyday medical practice.

The Universal Energy

When our bodies are in a healthy state we resonate with a rich and balanced flow of energy or life force. If this flow of energy is interrupted or thrown out of balance, illness occurs, or what is referred to as disease or dis-ease. Energy work, whether it involves the laying on of hands, magnets, prayer, acupuncture or breathing and relaxation techniques, all attempt to restore this healthy flow of energy to help bring the body back into balance with the universal life force that flows through all of us.

Some approaches break the body down into several energy centers called chakras while others deal with the body's overall energy field sometimes referred to as our aura. Still other methods use different terms in describing their approach but the underlying principles are the same, to bring back into balance the healthy flow of energy that permeates us all. The point is we are all tapping the same universal energy, albeit in different ways and on different levels, but it's the same life force.

I've heard many people refer to these approaches as New Age, which is somewhat of a misnomer because they more aptly could be called Old Age. Qigong (pronounced Chi-Kung) for example, is an ancient Chinese approach to health care that integrates physical postures with breathing techniques and focused intention in harmony with the universal life force, again, based on the same underlying principles. You can learn more about Qigong by visiting: http://www.nqa.org

On a biological level, our body is basically a highly evolved organism or mechanism that is made to heal itself. When we are in a healthy state our body can fight off all sorts of toxins it encounters in the environment. You can catch a cold with a fever and after a good night or two of rest wake up feeling all better without having done a thing. Your body will automatically fight off infections, heal cuts, bruises, and even broken bones. However, if your system is run down, you can become quite ill. Just like stress, the body can only take so much of it without some sort of relief or rejuvenation.

While going through chemotherapy, I met a famous Russian healer named Anatoly Kashpirovsky who had a positive affect on me. Like all great healers will tell you, they are not the ones doing the healing. It is your body healing itself. Dr. Kashpirovsky believes the body is embedded with a cellular memory of itself in a healthy state and can internally produce whatever drugs or chemicals are needed to restore the body to its previously healthy state. He claims to be able to influence this mechanism but is not the one doing the actual healing. That comes from within. Again, it's an ancient principle. As Hippocrates said, *Natural forces within us are the true healers of disease.*

I continued reading books by healers and famous psychics, such as Silvia Browne whom I had seen on television. Sylvia's books cover many topics including healing the body through spiritual methods and beliefs. In fact, one of the most powerful and sophisticated visualization techniques used for healing that I have ever tried is on page 213 in Sylvia Browne's book, *Adventures of a Psychic*. It is called *The Laboratory Technique* and begins with building a room in your mind's eye with specific details. Then, after acclimating yourself to the space and mentally placing yourself on a table in the room, Sylvia teaches you how to direct the universal energy to heal a specific ailment. It is an advanced technique that may require practice but it can be very effective and I highly recommend experimenting with it. Just like the breathing exercises, the more you work on it, the better it will work for you.

Reading Sylvia Browne's books and listening to her tapes also helped me to be more in tune to my own inner voice and intuition. This can help in deciding what sort of energy work to try because ultimately, you will have to gauge for yourself what works and with whom you are willing to work. **⚷ *My suggestion is to keep an open mind but learn to trust your intuition.***

Another great author and speaker on the subject of intuition is Caroline Myss, a medical intuit who has produced numerous books and audio tapes/CDs on intuition, including a four CD workshop called *Intuitive Power* which teaches you how to utilize your intuition for health and guidance. She also has a tape entitled, *Healing with Spirit* that is both fascinating and entertaining. It is an interview with Caroline Myss conducted by Michael Toms of New Dimensions Radio in which she talks about her history as a medical intuitive.

I recently came across another phenomenal book on intuition that I highly recommend entitled, *Diary of a Medical Intuitive* written by Christel Nani, RN, Ph.D. Christel started out as a trauma nurse in one of New York's busiest hospitals where through her intuition, she was able to accurately diagnose patients before the doctors. Eventually, she left to refine her skills and used them to help others heal. This book offers tremendous insight into the workings of a Medical Intuitive that I believe can help you better understand and utilize your own intuition.

– 10 –

Love and Prayer

"Some of the world's greatest feats were accomplished by people not smart enough to know they were impossible."

Doug Larson

Remember when your mother could make pain disappear with a loving kiss on the spot that hurt? When it comes to healing, the power of love cannot be underestimated. It can be more effective than any medicine available. I am not claiming to be an expert in this area, nor am I claiming to be an expert in prayer. However, like most things in life, I do believe the more you put into something, the more you will get out of it and with giving, the more you give the more you will have to give.

Love begins with oneself. As with maintaining a positive attitude, having a positive, loving self-image and a love of life in general will help boost your immune system. Again, it produces positive chemical changes in the body. In addition, I believe you cannot love and respect others if you do not love and respect yourself. In contrast, self-destructive behavior and self-hatred can break down your immune system and destroy not only you but anyone else around who cares about you. Whereas if you love and respect yourself, you will find others will love and respect you as well.

It is only natural at times while going through cancer treatments to feel sorry for yourself, especially when your hair starts to fall out. Not only is it emotionally painful, but when the hair actually falls out, your scalp will hurt. You will also probably feel tired and run down much of the time. It's hard to feel love under those circumstances. However, feeling too sorry for yourself or being overly critical of oneself can be detrimental to your health. Remember, positive thoughts and emotions will have a positive physical effect on your body and conversely, negative thoughts will have a negative effect. In order to heal, you will need to feel good about yourself. So, if you are overly critical and have difficulty loving yourself, I suggest doing something about it, and if necessary, seek counseling.

Continue listening to your audio tapes. You can also repetitively say positive affirmations to help put you back on track. For example, you can say things like, *I am loving and I deserve to be loved.*

Now here is where it gets interesting. In the aforementioned book, *Diary of a Medical Intuitive*, Christel Nani asserts that if you are not really sure about an affirmation, repeating it again and again won't work for you and the way to determine your level of belief is to say the affirmation out loud. If you don't feel your energy behind the words, you probably have your doubts. Christel offers a great way to solve this dilemma by simply adding acceptance of the conflict to your affirmation. For example, if you don't feel conviction in your voice when you say, *I am loving and I deserve to be loved*, you can add the words, *even if I'm not always sure I deserve it.* This is a great workaround that will increase the effectiveness of positive affirmations whenever you have reservations or self doubt.[7]

Another technique that can help you maintain a loving self-image is to try and bring back a loving moment in your past,

---

7 Christel Nani, *Diary of a Medical Intuitive* (2004) p. 58-64.

like the feeling of being head over heals in love. Try to recapture that feeling of walking on air. Take a deep breath and think of where you were, what music you were listening to, what time of the year it was. As the Righteous Brothers used to sing, *Bring back that lovin' feeling... Whoa that lovin' feeling...* There is simply no room for illness when you feel in love.

When love is in the air, everything feels better and you don't necessarily need a partner to experience it. You can love and cherish every moment that passes. Breathe in love with every breath you take. **⚷ *Fill your environment with love*.** Be passionate about your surroundings with all of your senses. Love can be found everywhere and as with joy and laughter, feeling love in your heart can produce endorphins that will help your body to heal.

I always liked the golden rule... *Do unto others as you would have them do unto you...* Try to love others as you would love to be loved yourself. As James Taylor sings, *Shower the people you love with love, show them the way you feel... things are going to work out fine if you only will...*

Praying to a higher order can also offer an infinite and powerful source of healing. It can provide great comfort and peace of mind. In fact, most people when faced with a serious illness or a loved one who is seriously ill, will turn to prayer. Even most non-believers will think of praying when facing death or a near death experience.

Praying and belief in God or some sort of higher order does not have to be based on a specific denomination. Nor does it have to be associated with a traditional father figure as in most western religions. It can simply be the belief in the universal energy or life force that is all around us.

Several studies have been conducted on prayer and its effect on healing, even the effect of prayer over great distances. One of the more compelling studies was conducted in 2001 and led by Mitch Krucoff, a cardiologist and director of interventional clinical trials at Duke. The study was inspired through observations made by Dr. Krucoff and his research team after visiting a hospital in India, where spirituality played an integral role. The team noticed that the patients in the hospital were much more comfortable and serene, which led to conducting a scientific study in the US, measuring the effects of spirituality on healing.

Dr. Krucoff said, *"Why a doctor would pray while his mother is in the OR, for example, can currently only be called intuition, maybe faith. Whether it actually makes any difference to the outcome of surgery is the kind of thing we're interested in studying scientifically."* [8]

The study was conducted with 150 men, all of whom were very ill. More than half had suffered a heart attack, most were former smokers, over a quarter had diabetes, over half had high blood pressure and all of them had been through a heart catheterization operation where a plastic tube had to be inserted into a coronary artery to reduce blockages.

These men were randomly divided into 5 groups. The first group received stress relaxation training, the second group received imagery training, the third group received therapeutic touch, the fourth group were prayed for by a variety of people from Baptists in North Carolina to Buddhists in Nepal, and the last group as the control, received no special treatment,

---

[8] http://www.prevention.com/article/0,5778,s-1-74-206-2029-2,00.html

other than the standard high quality of care offered at Duke. Neither the families, the patients nor the doctors knew who were being prayed for.

The doctors looked at two measurements, EEG readings and clinical outcomes, meaning whether or not any patients needed a repeat procedure, had a heart attack, developed congestive heart failure or died. As it turned out, the groups that received relaxation, imagery and touch had a 20 to 30% reduction in complications compared with the control group. However, the group that was prayed for had a 50% reduction in heartbeat abnormalities and a 100% reduction in clinical outcomes such as heart attacks and heart failure. Although Dr. Krucoff noted that the sample size was small, the results were suggestive and consistent.

Dr. Krucoff then raised funds for a larger study in 2005 that produced inconclusive results. Much like studying the effects of energy healers, this is an area where there are a lot of skeptics and those who just don't want to believe, regardless of how many people in the world claim to have been helped through the power of prayer. Skeptics will not be convinced until it is able to be proven definitively through scientific methods. The conundrum is that it may require a leap of faith in order for it to work. So again, you will have to use your own intuition and decide for yourself what works for you.

– 11 –

Healing Through Forgiveness

"Forgive yourself for your faults and your mistakes and move on."

Les Brown

From the start, I knew in order to completely survive cancer and to make sure it was never going to return I had to address the underlying causes, meaning how and why it began in the first place. After all, cancer is really the eating up of one's own body, so the body is literally destroying itself... a scary thought! If the body is really made to heal itself, what went wrong? Why did I get sick? What did I do to deserve it?

One of the issues I felt compelled to deal with was smoking. I was a heavy smoker prior to getting sick and there was a certain amount of guilt associated with it. I know that smoking dramatically increased my odds for developing lung cancer, but I had no way of knowing whether or not it was the sole reason. After all, there are smokers who never get cancer and people who develop lung cancer without ever smoking. Nevertheless, my smoking was now in the past and I couldn't change it, but I *could* change how I felt about it. I needed to let go of the guilt and I had to learn to forgive myself and move on.

I thought back to the points Louise L. Hay made in her book, *Heal Your Body: The Mental Causes for Physical Illness and the Metaphysical Way to Overcome Them*. She emphasized the emotional issues that cause cancer, such as deep hurt or longstanding grief or resentment. I wondered what issues I could have been holding that may have helped bring it on. I've always been a pretty happy guy and felt lucky, even when I wasn't so lucky. So, what could it be? As I gave more thought to this, instinctively, I felt it had to do with overall balance, that is, my being in true alignment of Mind, Body and Spirit. Although I had a healthy attitude about myself and about life, and I was now taking care of my body to the best of my abilities, I thought that maybe my spirit was somehow lacking, or diminished. Perhaps I had strayed from my mission in life and I had to get back on track, but I could not really put my finger on it.

I thought I could benefit from some sort of energy worker or a spirit healer, but I did not want to just go ahead and seek one out, especially with all the quacks in the field just looking to make money. I hoped one would come my way, or at least, I would get a solid referral or recommendation from someone I knew.

As I was trying to sort this out, a woman with psychic abilities and medical intuition came to me through a very trusted and skeptical source. This woman talked about me and said things that she should not have known, having never met me, so I was intrigued and decided to call her as she had offered. She was very wealthy and did not charge a penny for her help which put my own skepticism more at ease. When I called to speak with her over the phone, everything just felt right to me, so I took a chance and opened up.

She seemed to be more of a teacher or counselor than a healer, per se. We examined important relationships in my life such as family members and old friends. She told me that I had been harboring ill feelings and had to let these feelings go. In my heart, I knew she was correct but I did not know how to do it. She said it's easy. Just call them up and say, *Could you do me a favor? Would you forgive me for any unhappiness or anger that I may have caused you?* She said they might say something like, *Oh, you didn't cause me any anger*, or they might wonder what you are talking about, but don't worry, just follow it up by saying, *I just want you to know that I forgive you for any unhappiness or anger that you may have caused me.* Then get on with your life and try not to hold any anger or resentment again. They may not get it, and they may never get it, but I wasn't doing it for them. This was for me. In order to truly heal, I had to let go of past anger or unhappiness and move on. I had to forgive myself and forgive others.

Forgiveness is essential to spiritual health because holding on to old issues of anger and resentment will literally rot your spirit. Instead of living in the present, you will be exhausting your spirit on past hurts and angers that you must learn to let go of. This also includes old issues that you may no longer be consciously aware of as well as people with whom you are no longer in touch.

To help with this, she would say a prayer asking God to help me forgive those affecting me, in the name of the Father, the Son and the Holy Spirit. She also told me to pray for others to help them and to ask God to help me release any anger I might have. When I explained that I did not believe in the conventional sort of God that most people follow, we had a discussion about religion. I told her that I absolutely believe in a higher order, or divine spirit, but not the type of religious figure that people kill each other over. If God did not embrace every man, woman, child, plant and animal in the universe I was not buying into it. However, if I were to designate a God, it would be the universal energy, the life force and goodness that runs through all of us, and all living things. Mother Nature, if you will, the God and Goddess and goodness in all of us. She said if I understand that, then I understand God. Even though she referenced the Catholic tradition because of her own upbringing she acknowledged that God was non-denominational and recognized God as the divine force of life, assuring me that we were on the same wavelength.

I worked with this woman over a period of a couple of months and always on the phone. We would speak at least once or twice a week, sometimes more. This allowed me to reflect upon our discussions during my quiet times such as during my walks and while doing breathing exercises. It took me a while before I could get a handle on this and really be able to forgive myself. And whether I wanted to admit it or not, I was harboring a bit of anger over having contracted the illness to begin with. It tore apart my plans and almost took my life, but in order to truly heal, I had to be able to truly forgive myself and to truly forgive others because as she taught me, the way to heal is through forgiveness.

Changing habits of behavior takes practice because like most people, I have a tendency to slip backwards into old patterns of thought, especially concerning past issues, but she would hammer me sternly, as if I was not listening to her... I needed to let bygones be bygones and she made it clear that she was not going to be around forever to remind me. She was off to help other people. And she was right. This was something that I had to take charge of and I was the only one who could do it. There was no pill to take, no magic formula. It was something I needed to change in my thinking and it required work. So I picked up more audio tapes and books with positive affirmations to assist me in the process. Listening to them and reading them over and over helped me reprogram my mind by replacing negative thought patterns with positive thought patterns. It requires eternal vigilance and is something I am still mindful of to this day.

I recommend listening to *Healing with Spirit*, by medical intuit, Caroline Myss. She discusses how we rob ourselves of our spirit by negative thought patterns and by holding on to old issues and she offers ways to overcome it. I also recommend listening to Louise L. Hay's CD, *Cancer: Discovering Your Healing Power* that will help you to let go of these issues. It includes a guided meditation to help release any negative emotions.

We started in Chapter One by addressing our mind with the importance of a positive attitude, toward oneself and toward life in general. We also explored the concept of universal energy, and when that energy is flowing freely through us, we can allow that energy to restore our body to its previously healthy state. That is what our body is designed to do, and to be completely healthy and in balance, we need to be of sound mind, body and spirit. When we have a healthy attitude about ourselves and life, when we take care of our body and when we have a healthy spirit, we are at our optimum level of health.

Forgiveness, and letting your spirit thrive is an essential ingredient to your overall health and well being.

With practice, you will learn to do this without the tapes. When negative thoughts or situations arise, just calm yourself by taking slow, deep breaths. Allow the healing energy and life force to permeate your body. Close your eyes and fill your body with love. Think of a positive affirmation as you take deep breaths such as, *I lovingly forgive myself for any mistakes that I have made in the past and I lovingly surround myself with joy and happiness*, or, *I lovingly forgive whomever for any hurt or anger they may have caused me and I lovingly release any negative feelings over it*. You can tailor these anyway you would like and use whatever images or symbols work for you. ⚷ ***Just remember, you can help your body to reach its full potential and optimum state of health when you free your spirit from harboring ill feelings by healing through forgiveness.***

– 12 –

After Completing Conventional Treatments

"It's always too early to quit."

Norman Vincent Peale

You will probably be pretty tired after completing your treatments. The cumulative effect of chemotherapy and radiation therapy is not only physically taxing, but also emotionally draining. However, you should be proud of yourself. Have someone take your picture and date it. As the months pass, you will be able to see how far you have progressed.

When I first completed all of my treatments, someone said to me, *"Now comes the hard part."* I couldn't imagine what she meant but soon realized that the structure was gone... I didn't have to go in for any treatments. I did not even have to eat well. If I wanted to, I could fall into some of my old habits, working obsessively, eating poorly, smoking. It was actually easier to maintain my wellness program when I was going to the cancer center everyday. I was also facing the daunting task of trying to piece my life back together, one brick at a time.

The first and most important priority is to do whatever it takes to avoid allowing the cancer to return. Unfortunately, small cell lung cancer in particular has a way of coming back quickly and killing you, so it is imperative that you maintain a healthy lifestyle and continue to build up your immune system to guard against it. This can be done on a number of levels, physically, emotionally and spiritually.

Physically, you can make sure that you are eating and sleeping well. Continue to do the things that helped you build up your immune system. Allow yourself the time necessary to heal. Don't try to do everything at once. Remember, you can't do everything at once, but you *can* do something at once.

You may find that naps are helpful, even if you never were the napping type. ⌐ *Listen to your body and allow it to*

heal. It has been through a major shock and needs a break.

Try to maintain an exercise routine. Walking is always a good start. If the weather is too extreme, visit a shopping mall or find a treadmill to use. If you went through a lot of radiation to the lung, you will probably find that humidity is hard to deal with, especially at first. Try to stay in a dry atmosphere or air conditioned environment… and stay out of the sun. I was told to avoid direct sunlight for at least a year, especially on my head which sustained a lot of radiation. There is no need for an extra dose from the sun. Here again, you should be trying to minimize the amount of physical stress that your body has to overcome before devoting itself to your healing. Break up your day with exercises and periods of meditation. Scan your body to see if you are holding any tension and breathe through those areas to release that tension. Remember, your body was just put through the mill, so pamper yourself and give it a rest.

You may have developed certain allergies, even if you've never had them before. I developed a digestive disorder and without realizing it, went down the wrong road with a doctor who kept prescribing medications. My digestive system continued to get worse until I tried a gluten-free diet which solved the problem within days. It turns out I had developed an allergy to certain wheat products that I now can only eat in moderation.

Aside from physical issues, you may have more emotional issues to deal with than you realize. As discussed earlier, there is a psychological component to cancer that you should examine, and, if need be, look for a professional to address it with. What you want to avoid is falling back into the same patterns of behavior that helped bring about the illness to begin with. If you were all stressed out by obsessively working around the clock as I was, change your work habits. If you are sitting at a computer, take periodic breaks. Even small breaks for 30 seconds to stand up and stretch can be beneficial and change your focus. Repeat positive affirmations like, *I am going to maintain a sense of balance in my life*, or, *I will be patient and allow my body to heal.* Go out and buy a bright colored pad of Stickies and write yourself little notes to stick around the house and in your car. When you see one, slow down your breathing with deep, even breaths. Lower your shoulders and relax your jaw and facial muscles. Let go of any fear or anger and try not to become overwhelmed. I found a bumper sticker that I placed on a mirror indoors that reads, *Relax! You'll get there.*

Spiritually, do you feel that you are on the right path? How happy are you? Are you being true to yourself? Are you telling your loved ones that you love them? How fulfilling is your work? These are issues that you should be thinking about. If you are doing something that you feel is not your calling, or you are fulfilling someone else's idea of what you should be doing with your life instead of your own, you should reconsider. This may have been what brought on the illness to begin with and if you do not want it to return, you should be willing to examine everything and make whatever changes are necessary. After all, if you are not here, then nothing matters anyway. Think about it and seek advice if you are not clear.

After finishing months of chemotherapy and radiation, I did not want to be touched by any more doctors or nurses. I had been subjected to so many treatments and tests that I practically developed a phobia. Yet, I knew I needed some sort of body work to help me get back in balance.

One of the side effects I had suffered from the treatments was nerve damage, especially from my knees down. My feet felt as though they were asleep all of the time and they really hurt when standing barefoot on a hardwood floor. I also had strange nerve responses throughout my body. If I moved my head forward after any kind of exercise, I felt this spider web effect running through me and moving my head from side to side made me a little sick to my stomach. Some of this may have been from the chemo but more likely, it was due to the extra radiation I opted for to eradicate the tumor in my brain. However, I knew I could reverse it all given enough time, and I did. I just needed a little break before getting started.

I began taking vitamin B12 to help boost my energy and then started taking herb supplements like horse chestnut to help with the nerve damage in my legs. I did not think I could handle any heavy bodywork so after about a month, I started acupuncture treatments with someone I trusted and had worked with before. I felt it would be a good way to begin regaining a balanced flow of energy throughout my body. I also kept up with my breathing and visualization exercises and made sure I was eating and sleeping well.

The acupuncture treatments helped to an extent, but my feet were still a mess and I wasn't sure what to do. As luck would have it, a friend of mine told me about a wonderful reflexologist he had just met. Reflexology is much like acupuncture but without the needles. It works with pressure points on the feet (and hands) that correspond with various organs in the body. Acupuncture was a great way of balancing out my overall energy and reflexology worked directly on my feet, which steadily improved with each week that passed. It took over a year, but now my feet, head and legs are all back to normal.

Every three months, I would go back for a check-up which would include getting re-scanned. The first time, I didn't realize how much it would affect me, but as the day approached, I wasn't sleeping well and was emotionally on edge. Nevertheless, I would try to maintain a positive attitude and concentrate on taking slow deep breaths, especially in the doctor's office waiting for the results. What a relief it was to hear the doctors say the scans were good. I could literally feel the tension draining from my body.

On a couple of visits, there were small spots that appeared in my lung at a distance from where the tumor was located. This is not unusual and often due to the onset of a cold. However, the doctors wanted to be on the safe side by keeping an eye on it, and would have me return sooner rather than later. No matter how much they said not to worry, it would frighten me nonetheless. Fortunately, it would go away as predicted and I finally realized these visits were followed by a bit of a cold, hence the reason for the spots. Perhaps it was due to all the stress and fear that led up to these periodic scans. That's when I met the energy worker who suggested using visuals to dispose of fear, as discussed in Chapter Eight. So I worked at alleviating my fear and continued to improve my breathing and visualization techniques. I was better at it than ever before and I realized that once you teach your body to get rid of cancer, your body is smarter and if necessary, can make it go away again.

When someone would ask if the cancer was in remission, I would say, *No! It's not in remission. I am cured and I'm healthy again!* I never liked the term, in remission. It implies a temporary state of being. I beat this thing and I wasn't going to let it come back. Everyone has cancer cells in their body and under normal circumstances (with a healthy mind, body and spirit) the immune system keeps them at bay. It is when they multiply out of control that one becomes ill. Now, with more experience and knowledge than ever before, I feel better equipped to handle it and I really believe I will live a very long and healthy life as a result. It's like the old saying; *what doesn't kill you makes you stronger.* Nevertheless, I will always be more careful than I used to be.

After two or three years, my check-ups and scans became less frequent to the point where I'd go a year without being scanned, making it somewhat of a formality, but still a reminder of what could happen if I wasn't mindful. Then one day, I met an elderly woman who had survived a severe case of cervical cancer some thirty years before. I told her it had been about four years since I had completed my treatments and that I felt great, but at times I still worried that it might return. She calmly looked me in the eyes and said, *Eventually, you will realize that it's not about the illness anymore... It's about Living.* There was something in the way she said it that struck a chord in me and from that day forward, I let go of the cancer and *knew* I was healthy again.

Today, more than six years after completing my treatments, I no longer have to return for scans and any future check-ups are optional.

Postscript

So, *why did I survive* against all odds? I think doctors might credit the chemotherapy and radiation regiment. However, if that was the whole story, the survival rate would probably be much higher. I knew there had to be more to it than that. Somewhere between maintaining a positive attitude, being actively engaged in the decisions I faced, minimizing stress, eating well, breathing and visualization techniques, loving, laughing, prayer and forgiveness, in conjunction with the conventional treatments, I created a magical combination with help and guidance from the outside and orchestrated from within that brought me back to an optimum state of health.

It required more that just healing my body. I had to bring back into balance my Mind, Body and Spirit. With a healthy mental outlook on life, proper care and feeding of my body and a strong spiritual connection, I was able to reestablish a healthy flow of life force, the universal healing energy that resonates through all of us. As a result, I am now happy, healthy and still growing in mind, body and spirit.

⊶ *There is always something positive that can come out of a negative situation.* For me, cancer was a huge wake-up call and I sincerely believe that because of it, I am not only going to live a much longer and healthier life, but also a much happier and fulfilling one now that I am addressing the issues that I was not wise enough to address before.

I hope this book has inspired you and that it will help you to create your own magical combination that brings you back to your optimum state of health. If there is something in particular that has helped you, make sure you pass it on to others. Once you go through something like this, I believe you cannot help but want to help others. It is one of the most generous and therapeutic things you can do. Remember, the more you give the more you will have to give. So have fun living a long, healthy life with lots of love and joy!

Send comments to: ML@SurviveLungCancer.com

Additional Resources Available

THE AMERICAN CANCER SOCIETY – web site
http://www.cancer.org

NATIONAL INSTITUTE OF HEALTH – web site
http://www.ncbi.nlm.nih.gov

NATIONAL INSTITUTE OF HEALTH CANCER FAX
LINE – This is computer operated and can fax you all kinds of
information 301-402-5874

THE AMERICAN BOARD of MEDICAL SPECIALTIES to
check board certification of physicians 846-491-9091 or
http://www.abms.org

THE AMERICAN MEDICAL ASSOCIATION – You can
look up information on your doctors' training, etc.
http://www.ama-assn.org

STATE DEPARTMENT OF PUBLIC HEALTH – You can check your local Department of Public Health to see if there is anything negative about your doctor on file – Call Information

HEALTHFINDER – A government site that offers many links to helpful organizations http://www.healthfinder.gov

MEDLINE – A government database for looking up anything to do with health care where you can type in a question http://www.nlm.nih.gov

ALTERNATIVE HEALTH NEWS ONLINE – A great site for the latest information on alternative therapies http://www.altmedicine.com

ASK DR. WEIL – Another site for general information on anything to do with your health http://www.drweil.com

CENTER FOR ALTERNATIVE MEDICINE RESEARCH in CANCER University of Texas – A web site that evaluates some of the most controversial cancer treatments http://www.sph.uth.tmc.edu/utcam

HOLISTIC-ONLINE.COM – An all around site on alternative and integrative medicine and general nutrition http://www.holistic-online.com

HEALTH RECIPES.COM – Includes numerous articles and recipes for healthy eating

http://www.healthrecipes.com

HAY HOUSE, INC – A great place to find books, tapes and CD's on spiritual healing and wellness, including many that were recommended in this book http://hayhouse.com

HAY HOUSE RADIO – A free online radio station filled with shows on healing and spirituality, including archives of old shows by many of the authors mentioned in this book http://www.hayhouseradio.com

AMAZON.COM – The largest online bookstore I know of where you can search for new as well as used books on any subject http://www.amazon.com

You can also visit my web site: www.SurviveLungCancer.com for any updated information on this book.

NOTES